Adult Sleep Solutions:

Insomnia Solutions (100% Natural), How To Overcome & Reduce Stress & Anxiety, Effective Method, Without Drugs, Sleeplessness & Chronic Sleeping Disorder, Remedies, Relieve, Help

By Ed Austin

Introduction

Have you ever experienced difficulty in falling or staying asleep at night? Do you persistently wake up in the middle of the night, and cannot seem to go back to sleep again? If you have experienced these conditions, it is likely that you have insomnia.

Insomnia can be very disturbing and disruptive and can affect many aspects of your life. It is not easy engaging oneself in school and work after a number of sleepless nights. On top of that, because of the serious health risks that insomnia poses, it is important that one immediately seek medical help to cure insomnia.

There are pills, drugs, and other types of medication that might help a person get back to his or her normal sleeping habits, but there are effective, natural ways to cure insomnia, too. If you really want to have a good night's rest without the help of so-called chemical methods, then this book is for you.

This book contains proven steps and strategies on how to start getting a good night's sleep. It will help you restore your sleeping habits without having to resort to the use of drugs, pills, and other forms of medication. The methods you will find here are 100% natural and effective!

The first chapter will give you valuable information on insomnia, its causes, signs, and symptoms so you will be able to understand this sleep disorder better.

In the second chapter, you will learn about the importance of sleep and why it is necessary for one to have adequate sleep.

The third chapter gives suggestions on ways to change your habits as a cure to your insomnia.

The fourth chapter goes on by introducing to you various ways on how to become emotionally stable.

Ways on how to keep yourself relaxed can be found in the fifth chapter.

The sixth chapter begins by sharing to you the kinds of food that you should avoid and what to include in your diet to help you battle insomnia and achieve better quality sleep.

Finally, the book concludes by informing you of the risks and complications that may arise if your insomnia is untreated properly, much less left untreated.

Chapter 1 –
Insomnia and Its
Causes, Signs, and
Symptoms

Chapter 1 – Insomnia and Its Causes, Signs, and Symptoms

Insomnia is a disorder wherein a person finds it difficult to sleep at night, has difficulty staying asleep, or both. It is a condition in which a person experiences distorted sleeping habits. Insomnia is a sleeping disorder that needs to be addressed as soon as possible because it poses serious health risks that may affect many aspects of a person's life. But before proceeding to the natural, yet effective, ways to cure insomnia, it is first important to understand what insomnia is, its causes, signs, and symptoms.

This chapter will introduce to you information about insomnia, what causes it, and the conditions that a person will experience if he or she has insomnia. Knowing the causes, signs, and symptoms of insomnia will help a person identify effective measures that he or she should take in order to get rid of this sleeping disorder.

There are two types of insomnia. They are as follows:

1. *Primary Insomnia.* This type of insomnia is one in which a person is experiencing difficulty in falling asleep and/or staying asleep, but without a direct association to any health problems. It is a condition in which a person experiences sleeping disorder alone, without it being caused by other medical conditions.

2. *Secondary Insomnia.* The other type of insomnia is secondary insomnia. It is a

condition in which a person experiences a sleeping disorder, but with direct association to some health problems or medications. It can either be caused by depression, anxiety, asthma, heart problems, and other medical conditions.

Insomnia can also be classified according to how often it occurs and how long it lasts. The variations of insomnia are as follows:

1. *Acute Insomnia.* Acute insomnia is a short-term kind of insomnia. As the description suggests, it only lasts for a short period of time. Usually, this condition does not need immediate and serious medical attention, because it will just go away or cure itself after some time. However, it is still important to identify whether one's experience of acute insomnia could be a sign of other medical conditions.

Acute insomnia usually only lasts for a night up to a few weeks.

2. *Chronic Insomnia.* Chronic insomnia is a long-term kind of insomnia. As the name suggests, it lasts for a long period of time. This condition needs immediate medical attention because it can cause serious health problems if untreated. Chronic insomnia lasts for a month, or even longer.

Now that you are informed of the basic things you need to know about insomnia, the next important thing to understand are the causes of insomnia. What experiences or medical conditions could have led to the sleeping disorder that you are suffering from right now? Have you been really stressed out lately, or are there serious problems that have been bothering you? The following are the most common causes of insomnia:

Stress. Stress is one of the most common causes of insomnia. It is a feeling that one experiences when there are too many things that are bothering him or her, such as family problems, financial problems, pressing responsibilities at work and at home, dysfunctional and problematic relationship, and others. It can also be caused by feeling pressured to accomplish things that have to be done within a limited time. When one is stressed out, it may lead to problems and difficulties in his or her sleeping habits.

Environmental Factors. Insomnia can also be caused by environmental factors such as extreme temperature, noise, light, and other things that interfere with sleep. You might be living in an area where these things are prevalent and that is why you cannot seem to sleep properly.

Medications. The intake of certain drugs and medicines can cause insomnia. You might be taking pills and antibiotics to treat your cold, depression, asthma, allergy, and other health problems.

These medications can interfere with one's sleeping habits.

Emotional Problems. Things that make you feel terribly sad and depressed can cause you to experience difficulty in sleeping. You may have lost a loved one, or had your first breakup. You may be depressed because of a failing grade in school, or you are being bullied by your peers.

These experiences make you preoccupied, and will eventually affect your sleeping habits. You cannot seem to get these things out of your mind that is why you find it difficult to fall asleep and stay asleep.

How can one know if he or she is experiencing insomnia? The following are the signs and symptoms of insomnia:

Difficulty falling asleep and/or staying asleep. This is the main symptom of insomnia. You can easily say that you are suffering from insomnia if you experience this. There are also times when you will find it hard to get into a comfortable sleeping position. This is also a symptom of insomnia.

Sleepiness during daytime. Since you did not have enough sleep during the night, or have not had any sleep at all, you tend to become sleepy during the day. You do not feel refreshed, and you lack energy.

Difficulty concentrating. Insufficient sleep affects one's brain. Because of insomnia, you may find it difficult to concentrate on different things. You also experience problems with memory (i.e. becoming more forgetful and having a hard time remember things).

Now that you know the causes, signs, and symptoms of insomnia, you already have an idea of how difficult it is to lose sleep — it affects many aspects of your life. On the other hand, having adequate sleep is helpful and vital.

It is important to be aware of the importance of sleep and sleeping, so that you will be reminded that insomnia can be a serious health problem. The next chapter will share to you the importance of sleeping, and why it is necessary to have adequate, quality sleep.

Chapter 2 – The Importance of Sleep and Sleeping

Chapter 2 – The Importance of Sleep and Sleeping

Lack of sleep makes a person tired and weak throughout the day. He or she does not seem to have any energy at all do to his or her work, and to engage himself or herself in activities that he or she usually enjoys. Thus, knowing the importance of sleeping is important in making sure that you are having sufficient time to sleep, and that you will realize how important it is that you cure your insomnia immediately.

Sleeping helps a person improve his or her memory. Whenever a person is asleep, the brain processes the things that he or she learned during the day. He or she is unaware that his or her memory is already being sharpened while getting some snooze time. Science suggests that a person performs better on things that he or she learned during the day, after getting a good night's sleep. On the flip side, having inadequate sleep can lead to poor memory, or worse, memory loss.

Sleeping is also important because it prevents a person from having serious heart diseases. Researchers suggest that people who lack sleep are more prone to having high blood pressure and other heart-related diseases. These can pose a serious threat to the life of a person.

As the saying goes, "Prevention is better than cure." It is therefore important to sleep adequately in order to prevent these kinds of diseases, because acquiring these diseases is much more difficult to deal with.

Science has also discovered that having

adequate sleep makes a person more creative. This is a result of a more sharpened mind, and having more capability to think well. Sleeping can improve your performance in many aspects of life, including art. If you are also conscious about your weight, having enough sleep can be a solution. Adequate sleeping helps a person maintain a healthy weight. Lack of sleep can cause a person to be either overweight or underweight, but having just enough sleep helps you moderate your weight.

Sleeping also helps you be emotionally stable. It lowers your stress levels, and helps you to get rid of depression. Sleeping clears your mind from things that are bothering you, thus making you maintain a positive and healthy outlook in life.

Lastly, sleeping can keep you away from accidents. There have been many reported accidents on the road that were caused by sleepy drivers or drivers who have accidentally fallen asleep on the wheel. By having enough and adequate sleep, you will be able to have energy during the day, and be focused on whatever you are doing. This will keep you away from danger. In one way or another, sleeping may even help you save your life, your family's lives, and other people's lives.

Chapter 3 – The Natural and Effective Cure and Treatment for Insomnia: Changing One's Habits

Chapter 3 – The Natural and Effective Cure and Treatment for Insomnia: Changing One's Habits

Now that you know how important sleeping is, you should take immediate effective measures to cure your insomnia. One of the ways to cure insomnia without the use of drugs and medications is changing one's habits. This chapter will inform you of the habits that cause insomnia, and what you should do in order to change them.

If you are used to sleeping in the afternoon, or any time during the day, you should now learn to practice sleeping only at night. Taking naps during the day will only make you less sleepy at night. This will make it more difficult for you to fall asleep, and thus experience insomnia.

When it is already late, you should avoid alcohol, nicotine, and caffeine. These chemicals make your mind hyperactive, thus lessening the possibility that you will become sleepy at night. These are stimulants that will keep you awake, and you will find it very difficult to deal with them once they are already in your body.

Eating only a light snack before going to sleep may help you to have a good night's rest. Eating heavy meals for dinner may only cause you to feel uncomfortable because you are very full. It is enough that you go for a light snack. This will help you to become sleepy.

Although exercise is important, it is better to do it during daytime. Exercising before going to sleep stimulates your body, and it will make it more difficult for you to fall asleep. If you will be exercising at night, it is recommended that you do so three to four hours before bedtime.

As mentioned earlier, your environment affects your sleeping habits. Therefore, it is important that you make sure that your bedroom is comfortable to sleep in. Your bedroom must be well-lighted, free of noise, and the temperature must not be too high or too low. Science also suggests that there are certain scents that help a person fall asleep. Lavender, for instance, is considered a mild tranquilizer. If you have lavender oil at home, apply a small amount to your temples and forehead. As you smell its aroma, you will find it easier to fall asleep.

Researchers have also discovered that exposure to natural and artificial light affects one's sleepiness. If you are more exposed to natural light during the day, there is a greater possibility that you will be sleepy at night. Increased exposure to artificial light, however, reduces the possibility of becoming sleepy. Thus, it is important that you expose yourself more to natural light than to artificial light.

If you are a workaholic, it is recommended that you manage your time for work properly. Working at night can disrupt your sleeping habits. Maintain the same sleeping habits as much as possible. Avoid irregular shifts at work as much as possible, and finish your work during daytime.

Taking a warm bath before going to bed can help one to become sleepy. Bathing will make you feel comfortable and relaxed. Relaxation is the most influential factor that could lead to sleepiness. If you are perfectly comfortable with yourself and with your environment, it will be easier for you to fall asleep.

Breathing practices and meditation can also help you ease your mind and body and prep yourself to sleep.

These things will all be helpful in making you sleepy at night.

Regulate your sleeping time. Make it a point to be at bed at a certain time every night. This will condition your mind and body to become sleepy once that time nears. Research has shown that it takes 21 days for something to become a habit, so stick to your designated bedtime for 21 consecutive days.

These are just some of the habits that you need to practice to make becoming sleepy easier for and come naturally to you. However, improper habits are not the only reason that people encounter sleeping difficulties. Another factor could be emotional problems. Whenever a person is bogged down by negative thoughts, he or she could not just seem to stay asleep for the rest of the night. This problem will be addressed in the next chapter. It will inform you of tips and techniques on how to manage emotional pressures.

Chapter 4 – The Natural and Effective Cure and Treatment for Insomnia: Dealing with Emotional Pressures

Chapter 4 – The Natural and Effective Cure and Treatment for Insomnia: Dealing with Emotional Pressures

Being very depressed about a lot of things can be one factor that could account for why you find it difficult to sleep. For example, you may have received a phone call informing you of the death of a loved one. Or maybe you were scolded by your boss at work because you came in late. Or maybe when you got home from work, you had an argument with your husband, and he kept shouting at you. These things could all invade your thoughts, and it is natural for you to find it difficult to get rid of them. This chapter will share to you some tips on how to manage and neutralize your anxiety that could eventually bring back your normal sleeping habits.

You usually feel terribly sad and worried whenever your mind is filled with negative thoughts. To manage emotional pressures, it is important that you maintain a positive outlook in life. There may have been bad things that have happened to you lately, but keep in mind that things will get better in time. Thinking positive thoughts will help you calm down and keep yourself at ease. When you have already mastered this trick of thinking positively, negative thoughts will no longer keep you up at night.

Talking to someone close to you will be helpful. Sometimes, your emotions need an outlet for you to feel less pressured. Ask him or her for advice that could help you with your problem. A friendly and encouraging conversation with a person you can trust can help you make those emotional negativities go away. You can phone a friend before going to sleep, or pop by your sister's bedroom before you take a rest in your own. Welcome humor and keep the conversation light, but motivating. After doing this, you will feel more at ease and free from troubled thoughts.

Meditation and breathing exercises will also help you to stay at ease. When meditating, just let your thoughts fly and release everything through your breathing. Take deep breaths once in a while to release depression and negative thoughts. Make this a habit every night, before you go to bed, so that you will be able to stay comfortable and relaxed as you take a good night's rest.

Lastly, take everything slowly. Resolve your problems one after the other. Do not pressure yourself to resolve them all in one go. Be patient and understand that things will unfold naturally if you will just let them. By doing so, your mind will be free from emotional pressures.

Now that you know the things that you need to do to condition your habits and your emotions, the next important thing is to be informed of different relaxation techniques. These tips and techniques will be introduced to you in the next chapter.

Chapter 5 – The Natural and Effective Cure and Treatment for Insomnia: Relaxation Techniques

Chapter 5 – The Natural and Effective Cure and Treatment for Insomnia: Relaxation Techniques

One of the factors that can cause sleeping problems is the inability to relax. Usually, the reason some people find it difficult to fall asleep, or to stay asleep for the rest of the night, is that they are unable to keep themselves relaxed. This chapter will introduce to you several natural, yet effective, tips and techniques to keep yourself relaxed before sleeping, and even when you suddenly wake up in the middle of night.

One of the ways to relax is to do abdominal breathing or taking deep breaths. People take only shallow breaths most of the time. Breathing deeply and fully will make and keep you relaxed and at ease. This can be done by breathing not only through your abdomen and chest, but also through your ribcage, belly, and your lower back. Before you go to sleep, close your eyes and slowly take deep breaths. It will be much more effective if you make the next breath deeper than the last. Inhale through your nose, and exhale through your mouth. Abdominal breathing requires that you practice it regularly so that you will master this relaxation technique.

Another way to keep you relaxed is through progressive muscle relaxation. This is a relaxation technique in which you tense your muscle first before finally relaxing it. The trick is to lie down comfortably and tense the various muscles of your body, starting from your feet and then going up. After holding the tensed muscle for 10 to 15 minutes, slowly relax them. After doing it to the muscles in your feet, proceed to the other parts of your body until you reach the top of your head. After you have done this to your entire body, you will be able to relax. Similar to abdominal breathing, this technique also requires that you practice it regularly.

Lastly, meditation is a truly effective relaxation technique. As mentioned in the previous chapter, this can be done by just letting your thoughts fly while breathing deeply and slowly. Release all your thoughts, especially the negative ones, as you exhale. Make this a part of your bedtime routine, and in no time, you will no longer find it difficult to relax and fall asleep at night.

Now that you know the tips and techniques on how to relax and keep yourself relaxed before going to sleep, the next step is to make sure that you have a healthy diet. See to it that those kinds of food do not disrupt your sleeping habits. It is also important to include in your diet the kinds of food that are helpful in making you sleepy at night. Information about the necessary changes in your diet will be discussed in the next chapter.

Chapter 6 – The Natural and Effective Cure and Treatment for Insomnia: What to Include in Your Diet

Chapter 6 – The Natural and Effective Cure and Treatment for Insomnia: What to Include in Your Diet

There are certain kinds of food that could either be helpful or disruptive to your sleeping habits or sleep schedule. This chapter will inform you about the kinds of food that you should avoid, as well as the kinds of food that you should include in your diet, so that you will eventually have no more difficulty in falling asleep and staying asleep at night.

A brain chemical that helps a person sleep is serotonin. Serotonin can be produced by an amino acid called tryptophan. Therefore, it will be helpful that you consume foods that have tryptophan in them.

Examples of these are turkey, chicken, and banana. Eating small amounts of this food before going to sleep will be helpful in making you sleepy. Be reminded that you should not eat too much food before going to sleep. Taking heavy meals at night is not advisable by health experts. Small amounts are just enough.

It is easier for this amino acid to enter the brain with the help of carbohydrates. Just like when you were still a child, make it a habit to prepare a glass of warm milk paired with a piece of cookie (one that is not too sweet, though) or mixed with a spoonful of honey. Make sure that the milk has tryptophan in it. After finishing this small snack, the carbohydrates will help the amino acid get into your brain, helping you to find it easy to fall asleep.

There are also some kinds of food that you have to avoid. Spicy food before bedtime is a bad idea. The spices that these kinds of food contain can irritate your stomach. You will find it more difficult to fall asleep, because you are in pain — it will only cause you to become very uncomfortable. Even if you managed to fall asleep, these spices will wake you up in the middle of the night. Intake of sweets is also not advisable. Sugar can make a person feel jumpy and is a known stimulant. Because of this, it will be much more difficult to fall asleep. If you really cannot resist your sweet tooth craving, make it a point that you take your sweets three to four hours before you go to sleep so that they will be properly digested by then.

After identifying the kinds of food that you should avoid and the kinds of food that you should include in your diet to help you maintain a normal sleeping habit, the next thing is to combine all these with all the other tips, tricks, and techniques that you have learned in the previous chapters. Make sure to practice them regularly and in no time, you will no longer encounter sleeping problems. However, if you do not do anything about your insomnia, you may experience more serious health conditions. You will find out more about these risks and complications in the next chapter.

Chapter 7 – The Various Risks and Complications of Insomnia

Chapter 7 – The Various Risks and Complications of Insomnia

If not addressed properly, insomnia can lead to more complicated problems. As mentioned in the earlier chapters, insomnia poses health risks that may affect not only your body, but also the other aspects of your life, including your relationships with other people. How much worse can insomnia get? What happens when one does not treat his or her insomnia properly and seriously? This chapter will warn you about the possible risks and complications that insomnia brings.

Aside from the greater possibility of getting yourself involved in an accident, insomnia imposes serious health risks. Memory, thinking, and learning abilities are just some of the many aspects of your health that can be affected if you allow your insomnia to remain untreated. These kinds of problems do not only make it difficult for you to process your thoughts and ideas; they also make you incapable of making the right decisions, and taking the proper actions. Your thoughts become distorted and you will have a hard time thinking properly since were not able to get adequate sleep.

Inadequate sleep can also lead to problems in your immune system. Despite being protected with vitamins and other medicines, your immune system will no longer be able to respond properly to vaccinations. In addition, researchers have discovered that losing sleep makes you more vulnerable and more sensitive to pain. As a result, this will cause you to feel discomfort, and eventually lose sleep once again.

Insomnia can lead to serious diseases such as diabetes. By not having adequate sleep, your body cannot respond well to insulin. Because of this, insulin resistance occurs and leads to diabetes. High blood sugar levels can also result from not having enough hours of sleep. This can complicate diabetes or raise your risk of getting diabetes. And if this happens, there is a greater risk of developing heart diseases and hypertension as well. Increased inflammatory response is one of the effects of insomnia, and this contributes to he greater possibility of encountering heart problems. So, if not treated properly, these diseases can even pose a serious risk to one's life.

Another thing that can arise from insomnia is

obesity. Science suggests that when a person loses sleep, he or she has a greater tendency to resort to eating very heavy meals. Because of the changes in the levels of hormones, people who lose sleep are not able to regulate their appetite and food intake. When a person eats too much, he or she will gain weight. And when a person gains too much weight, this can lead to obesity, which also poses a great risk to one's health.

These are the different risks and complications that you may encounter if you leave your insomnia untreated or if you do not take your sleep disorder seriously. Aside from poor performance at work, lack of sleep causes diseases that can be life-threatening. You should not wait for these diseases to arise before you consider curing your insomnia through natural ways.

Conclusion

Hopefully, after reading this book, and practicing the tips and techniques it contains, you will no longer experience any difficulty in falling asleep and staying asleep at night. You will be able to enjoy more nights with adequate and quality sleep.

These tips, tricks, and techniques in this book may not involve the use of drugs and medications, but they are equally effective. If you regularly do these practices and techniques, you will be able to get rid of your sleeping disorder, and you may also keep yourself away from diseases that can affect your health.

Thank you again for reading.

I hope you are on your way to a good nights sleep.

www.ingramcontent.com/pod-product-compliance
Lightning Source LLC
Chambersburg PA
CBHW070411190526
45169CB00003B/1210